Workout:

30 Interval Workouts To Do Anytime and Anywhere

The information herein is offered for informational purposes solely, and is universal as so. The presentation of the information is without contract or any type of guarantee assurance.

The trademarks that are used are without any consent, and the publication of the trademark is without permission or backing by the trademark owner. All trademarks and brands within this book are for clarifying purposes only and are the owned by the owners themselves, not affiliated with this document.

Table of Contents

* * * * * * * * * * * * * *

Introduction: Fitting Health into Your Schedule

We all live off of a busy itinerary. From the moment that you wake up in the morning you have a ton of things that you have to do. You need to get your children to school and yourself to the office. You have bills to pay and moves to make. You have seemingly endless tasks and chores that need to be taken care of, and a very limited time frame in which to do them. By the end of the day you are lucky if you even remember that you had planned a workout as part of your routine, let alone actually working out!

This is the kind of pattern that we find ourselves in every single day, in which we can't even seem to squeeze in that extra half hour for a brief jog or session in the weight room. And each time you chastise yourself and promise to do better, but each time you end up failing miserably and ultimately questioning whether or not you will ever find the time to lose those extra pounds!

And then, in this inevitable spiral, the excuses begin to mount as well as the pounds. With these caked on pounds come the guilt, and the cycle of despair repeats! But if you can just set aside ten minutes at various intervals throughout the day you can change your life and break out of this negative tailspin for good! Let this book change your whole fitness routine, and allow you to finally fit health into your schedule!

Chapter 1: Getting Started with your Routine

In starting out this workout regimen with you, I really don't think it's my place or necessary to start lecturing you about why it is that you need to develop a good health routine. The very fact that you are reading this book right now is testament enough to me that you are already motivated to improve how healthy you are. Even if you don't want to lose weight, even if you are as skinny as can be, there are still plenty of reasons that you should increase fitness in order to improve cardiovascular health and enhance your muscle tone.

There are many reasons to get healthy besides weight loss and a high intensity, interval based workout is a great way to create that sense of health. This kind of workout routine is perfect for people with busy schedules because it can be adjusted in order to fit the individual's routine and capabilities. These exercises take just 10 minutes to complete, and in order to do them spaced out throughout the day, you can set your alarm/timer so that it goes off at approximately at 18 different intervals a day, letting you know to begin your routine.

If it helps you can also switch your timer to stopwatch mode, so that you can be as precise as possible. Each it one of these workouts should really take no longer than ten minutes. This is why it is so important to time them! With an accurate timing mechanism you can make all the difference in the world. This is the best workout for the busy person! It just takes a moment to kick start your whole routine!

Chapter 2: The Best Workouts for your Time

There are many workouts that you could do in a short amount of time, but this chapter is going to demonstrate some of the best that you could do without wasting any of that precious moment by moment commodity! Having that said, we all need a way that we can work out quickly and efficiently. So here it is; the best workouts that *do not* waste your time!

<u>*Air Squats*</u>

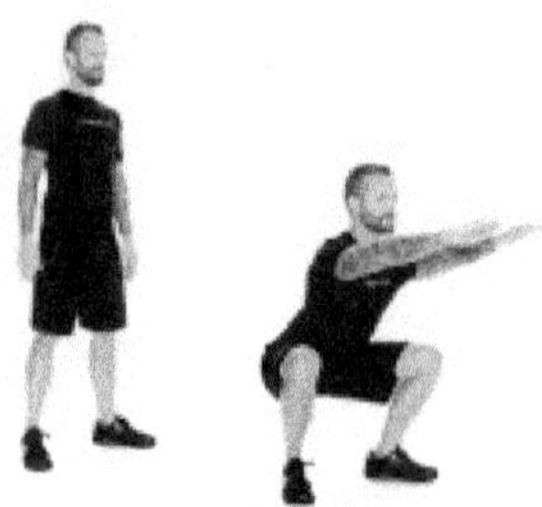

For this exercise you are going to want to stand up with your feet at hip width apart. Next, pull your shoulders all the way back so that you can focus on the core of your torso. After you have done this, now focus on putting your buttocks and hip toward the ground as if you were about to sit down. Basically put yourself in a sitting position while you squat in mid air. The way I usually describe this maneuver to people is that they should be pretending to sit down in an invisible chair.

At least that sure beats the way my original instructor told me was a bit more graphic, he said to pretend you are squatting and using the bathroom! Not exactly a fun thing to visualize with thirty other people in a workout class! So yes, let's just stick to the program here folks! And pretend you are sitting on an invisible chair! And as you imagine yourself sitting down on your chair, focus on keeping all of your weight firmly planted on your heels. As you sit, move yourself down until your upper legs become parallel to the floor, and lift your arms up in the air as you move downward. Get ready to feel the burn!

Burpees

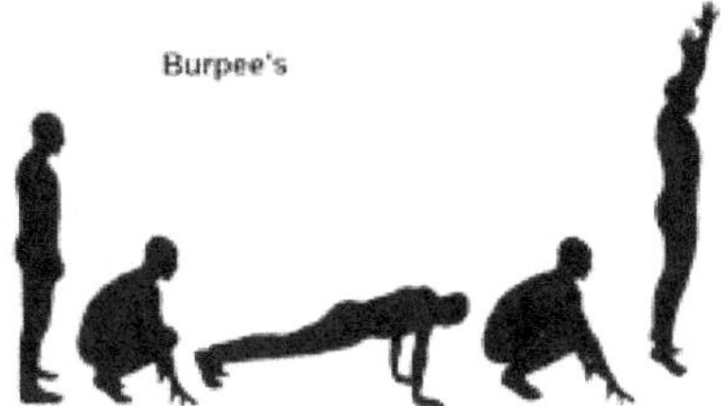

The Burpee is a great workout for anyone wishing to get right to the point of exercise, toning up and burning calories! Ok, to do this one guys, you are going to need to get into yet another squatting position. It doesn't sound pretty, but pop a squat folks! And just like you did for your air squat, except this time place your hand right in front of you on the floor. After this you can put your feet back toward a pushup pose. Next, put the feet back in place in your squat pose.

Finally, you will then break it all up by jumping straight up into the air and clapping your hands together, like some kind of an unfulfilled jumping jack! Get ready to go Burpee guys! The burpee is great because it works out your chest, as well as activating your hamstring and abdomen muscles. It manages to work the whole body in just a few signature moves, greatly burning fat in the process. I have to admit, I do love my burpee!

<u>***Dive Bomb Pushup***</u>

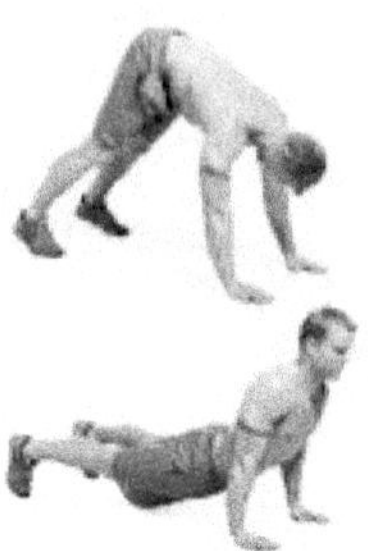

To begin you will go down into the move infamous to yoga fanatics around the world, known as the "downward dog". This is the pose in which you take on a form similar to a dog bending forward. Do this by putting your toes and hands on the floor while you push your back up into the air, and position your chest down toward the ground. Once your entire body is contorted into this position, take a moment before bending your elbows and dropping down into your first pushup.

The dive bomb is a great way to work all of the core muscles of your body. Just do this well simple, well balanced, and well placed exercise during one of your ten minute work out routines and it will make all of the rest of your day a whole lot easier! So don't forget to do your dive bomb push ups folks!

Handstand Pushups

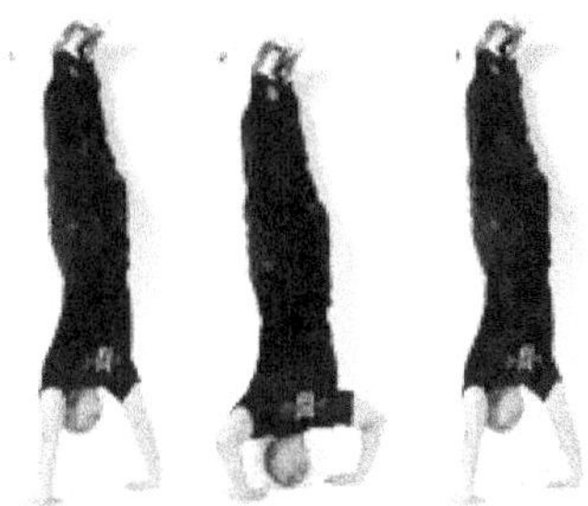

Doing pushups while standing on your head is one of the most vigorous workouts you could ever do in such a short amount of time. But I realize that for many of us standing on our hands may be a feat easier said than done. Some of you have probably never stood on your hands in your life. So taking that into consideration, if you never have done this before, one of the easiest ways to get started is to use a wall for support. Practice hanging yourself upside down, while kicking your legs up against the wall for extra traction.

The wall itself will work as your safety net to keep you from falling down. As you gain more confidence in your hand stand. Once you have achieved your hand stand just lower yourself down slowly toward the ground by bending your elbows, stay for a moment, and then begin pushing back up and repeating. This exercise is great for working out your gluteus maximus, abs, and upper leg muscles. Do it as many times as you can during the ten minute interval and you will have quite a workout indeed. So get ready to take a stand for fitness—a hand stand that is!

High Knees

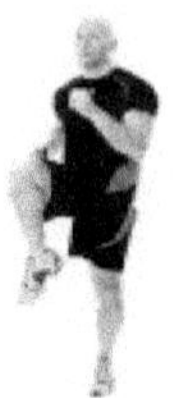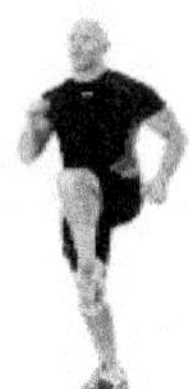

For this one all you have to do is stand in place with your feet spread wide apart. Then move your right knee in toward your body, and then quickly lower your leg to the ground. Do this with your left knee about ten times and then switch it up by doing this exercise once again with your right knee. After you have done that you can then alternate back and forth as much as you want. You could also throw in a rope in order to turn this exercise into a kind of jumping-rope routine. This exercise isn't called "high knees" for nothing. It is the high knee thrusts that make this such a great and enriching part of your workout routine.

Jump Lunges

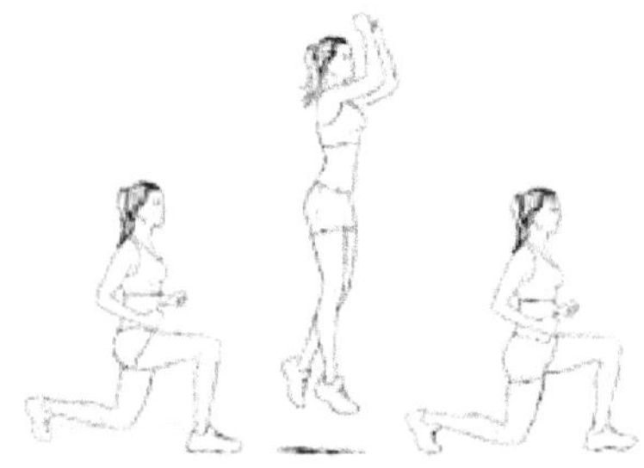

Providing a great cardiovascular workout, jump lunges can be an important part of your 10 minute workout routine. Begin this exercise by positioning your right foot in front of you, and your left foot behind. From this stance then begin to start bending each knee until you are in a kind of squatting position. While doing this, just make sure that your right foot is parallel against the ground with the knee of your right leg so far down that it is nearly scraping the ground.

Now put your arm behind you (doesn't matter which arm) and move it to a 90 degree angle. Once you are in this position, now you can lunge forward in a rapid, advancing movement. You start this one out in a lunge position and then with your knees reaching down to the floor you can then repeat the move so that you can keep up with this exercise for the full ten minutes. Now you can switch everything up by jumping back in rapid succession, with your leg pushing back and forth. You can then repeat this as much as you can.

Mountain Climbers

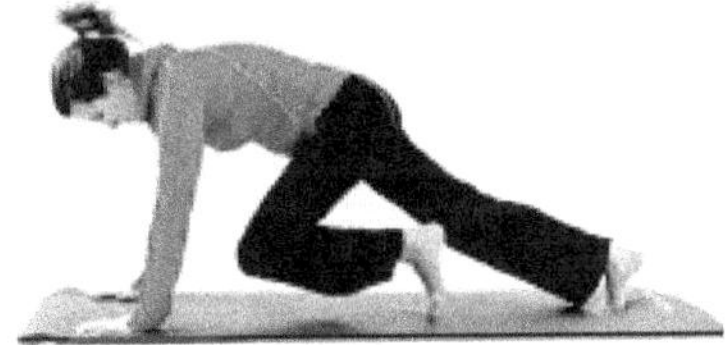

To do this one, start out in the push up pose, as if you are getting ready to do a round of push ups. You can then move your knees in quick succession up to your chest, as if you are running. Basically with this exercise you are simulating what would really happen if you were running up the side of the mountain. So as you could imagine, just as you would expend a lot of energy going up the sheer cliffs of a mountain range.

For this ten minute exercise you will also burn a lot of calories in a short period of time from the vigorous movements involved in your simulated climb. This exercise is great for getting a bounce in your heart rate. When you do it, just make sure that your back is pointed toward the ceiling, one leg is folded up in front of you, tucked into your chest, and alternate the leg that you use.

Pike Jumps

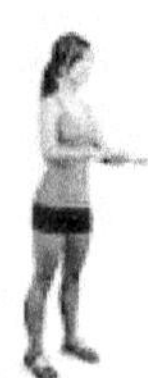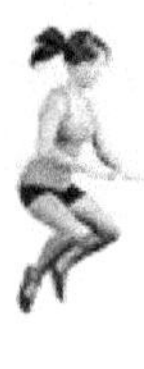

In order to do Pike Jumps, you can start out in the downward dog position, once you do this you can then pop up back on your feet and land on the other side. The rest of this is then just basically a "rinse, wash, repeat" and you are good to go! Now you can switch to the other side, in order to strengthen your entire core while you twist and try to keep in rhythm during this challenging ten minute, interval exercise.

Pistols

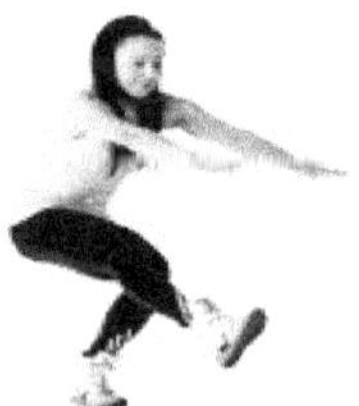

In this exercise you will stand up on one leg and then keep your other leg parallel to the floor. Now slowly pull yourself down to the floor as if you are attempting to sit down on the ground. You can then push down to the ground as much as possible and get your thighs down to the ground. Being able to squat on just one leg presents itself as a major challenge.

It is not only difficult to maintain your balance; it is also quite a challenge just to have enough muscle strength to be able to lift yourself off of the ground. This one move manages to activate your core like no other; igniting your hamstrings, and calves, as well as your gluteus maximus. This workout is a must have for your ten minute work out routine.

Pushups

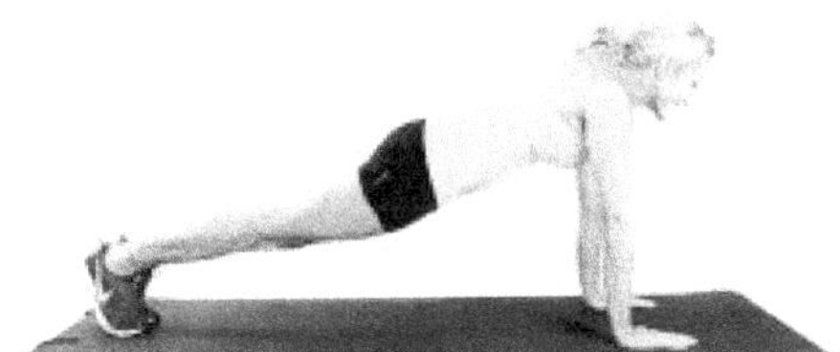

Anyone that ever had high school gym class remembers this simple but sweat breaking exercise. Pushups are a workout that you can easily do within a ten minute time frame. To get started, put yourself in that basic position stretched out to your full length, face down with toes and hands on the ground. Now just do what comes natural and push yourself up, back and forth as much as possible. This little routine will work to tighten your gluteus maximus, thighs, and abdominal muscles.

<u>Reptile Push Up</u>

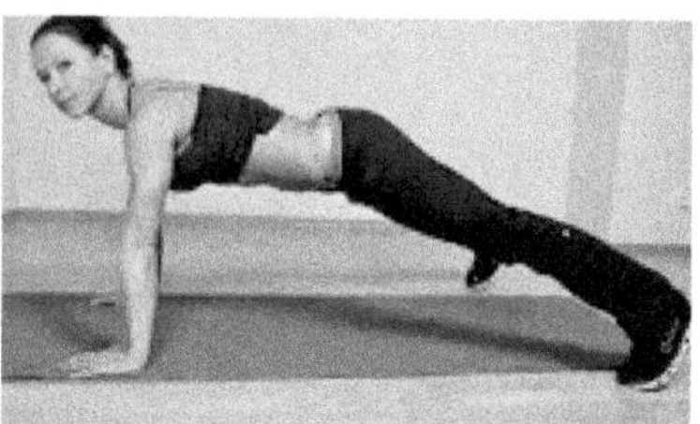

This one is basically a variation of the regular push up. Just tart out with your shoulders positioned right above your palms. Now tighten your thighs, glues, and abs. Now lower your chest down to the floor, and brig your knees up to your arms, so that you can finish the routine. Now just repeat as much as you can within your allotted ten minute time frame. You don't have to be a reptile in order to enjoy this quick ten minute exercise! So get ready to do your reptile push ups! You won't regret it!

<u>Sit Ups</u>

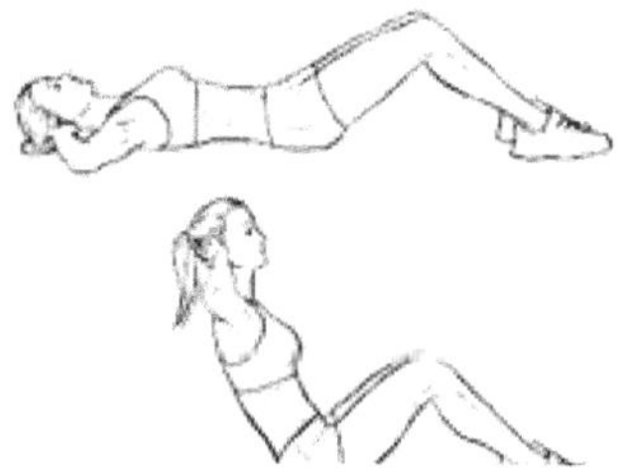

In order to do your sit ups you will lay on the ground with your legs spread out in the butterfly position. Now stretch your arms our in front of you, and use your abs to pull yourself up off of the floor. Then just reach out to your two feet with your fingers, allowing you to continue the motion of your chest. This is a classic exercise that will keep you in shape for as long as you do them! Sit ups are always a great addition to your ten minute workout routines.

<u>*Squat Jumps*</u>

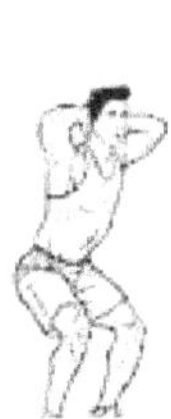 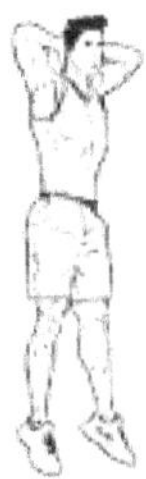

In order to do squat jumps, you have to stand with your feet about a shoulder length width apart. Now you can move yourself down into a mid-air sitting position, lined up with the direction of the floor. Hold this pose for a few moments and then jump up out of it as fast as possible. This is your squat jump!

After landing from this jump, simply repeat the process, and engage in your squat jumps as much as possible. Make sure that you are standing with your feet at least shoulder width apart when you do this one, and then simply jump up as hard and fast as you can, making sure that once you land you are right back in the same squat pose once again.

<u>*Tuck Jumps*</u>

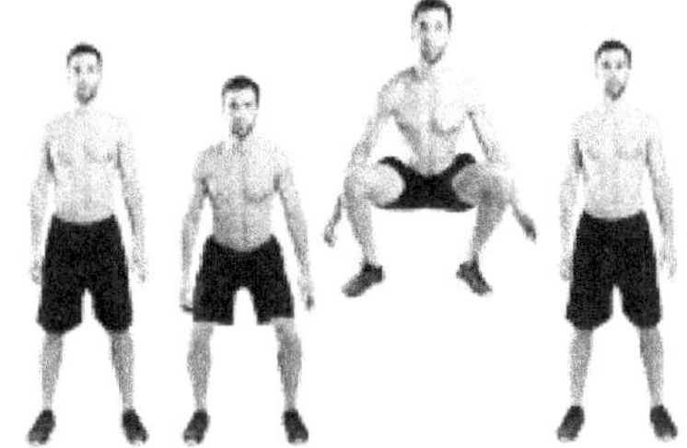

For Tuck Jumps you will need to take on a wide stance about shoulder width apart. Now jump up as much as possible, bringing your knees to your chest, with your back held upright. This is a high intensity, short burst kind of work out, so you really need to make the most of it.

This exercise is used quite a bit by basketball and soccer players who wish to improve their jumping ability, because this one simple move does much to strengthen your legs and the whole lower core of your body. After doing a tuck jump, once you land, just repeat this as much as possible within your ten minute window.

V Ups

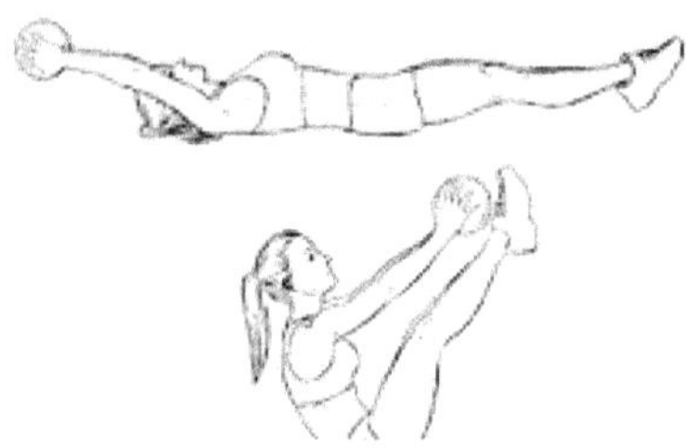

To get started on this one, lay down on your back, and then stretch out your arms above you, making sure that your legs are as straight as possible. You want to extend your body to its full length. When I do this, I usually imagine myself being a cat stretching out on its back in the sun, but just use whatever imagery works for you! While you are doing this you need to raise up your hands and feet as much as possible, keeping them in solid alignment.

Walking Lunges

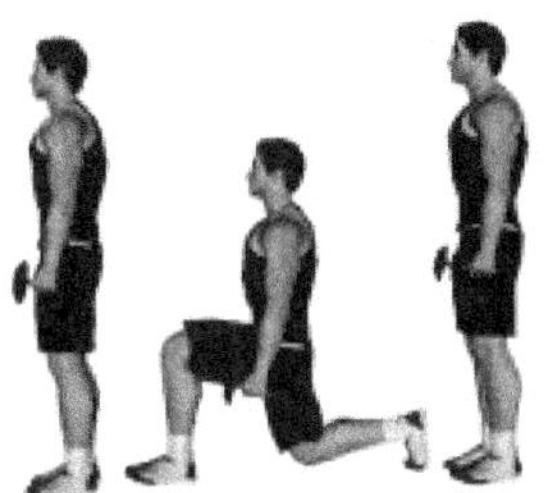

As you get started on this one you need to be in a lunging pose, which means that you will have your knees to where they are almost touching the floor. Now without even taking the time to pause, you need to alternate your legs, and move ahead into an all out lunging position. From here you can continue in your leg alterations, and repeat as many times as necessary within your ten minute time frame.

Chapter 3: More Workouts to Keep You in Your Routine

In this chapter we will deal with all of the other workouts that you can do in order to keep you focused and dedicated on your routine. It is really important to keep your metabolism going, you can do this by rigorous exercise and calorie burn in ten minute intervals. Here are a few examples that could really build upon and help your overall routine.

Clockwork

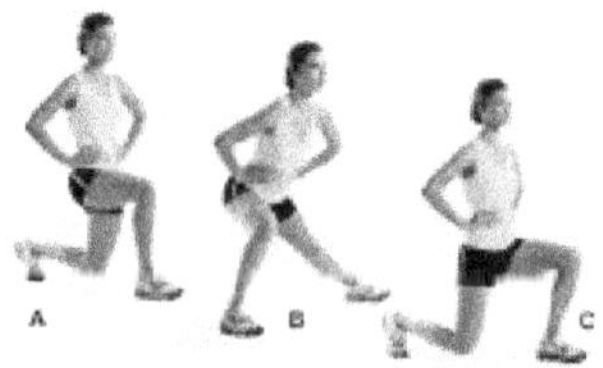

This workout has a name that says it all! "Clockwork" keeps you in time and is a great way to regulate your metabolism. Just stand with your feet together. Put your left foot forward, this will be known as the 12 o' clock position. This will take you about 3 feet, and then you can bend your knees and work your core into a lunging movement. This will allow you to keep the front portion of your knee behind your toes.

Now, without leaning forward, press your left foot in, as you rise up from the ground with your feet together. Now just move your left foot out from your side, and keeping your feet apart at the hips, bend your knees and bend your hip so that you can squat with your knees behind your toes. Finally just lower back into your lunge and then rise again. The rest is simply one great big, "rinse, wash, and repeat".

One Legged Lunges

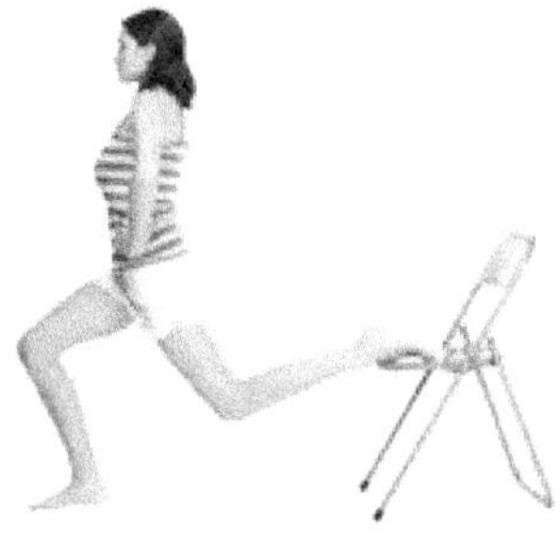

This is no ordinary lunge my friends! Because by just simply elevating one foot up in the air behind your, you can use this leg to gain extended leverage and really work out your other leg! Just bend this knee and allow yourself to lower into a classic lunge pose. Now you can move the front of your knee behind your toes and press it into your foot so that you will be able to stand yourself back up again and gain traction, and a great workout in the process! Do these one legged lunges as much as you can within your allotted ten minute intervals.

Monster Squats

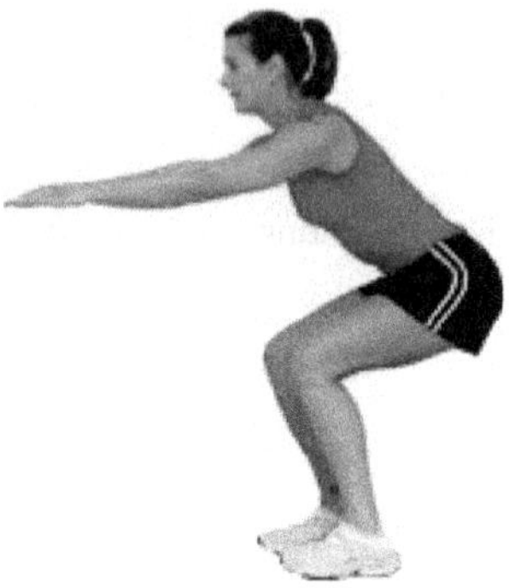

This exercise is the beast! In fact it is a monster! Monster squats allows you to work out your thigh and the muscles of your gluteus maximus like no other! And in quick succession! In order to do this exercise, you just need to stand with your feet wide apart, at about shoulder width, with your toes pointing out and your arms relaxed.

Now simply stand up and begin to feel that burn! You will then feel it again as you start raising your left knee up in the air. Finally place your footing back on the ground and you will be able to lower it into the next squatting pose just by raising your other leg. These squats are a monster of a workout and they will keep you very busy throughout your ten minute intervals.

Arm Sculptor

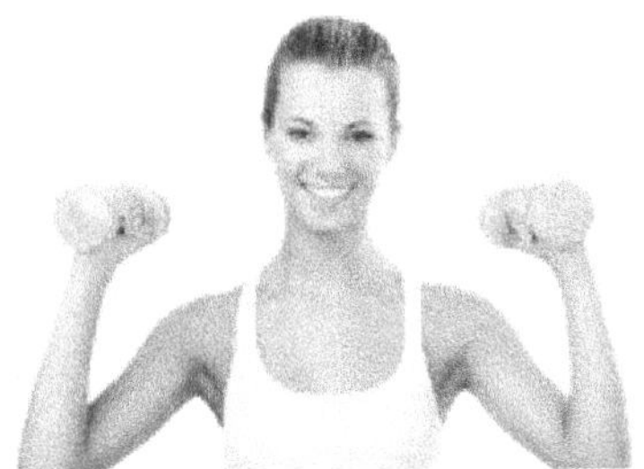

By doing this you can exercise you can really sculpt your arms! This one is designed for you to be able to make swimming motions while standing in place so that you could move your arms as if you are just going for a swim. Repeat this arm sculptor as much as you want. This is a great exercise to activate all of the muscles within your arms as you sculpt them into their best shape!

Side Plank Push Ups

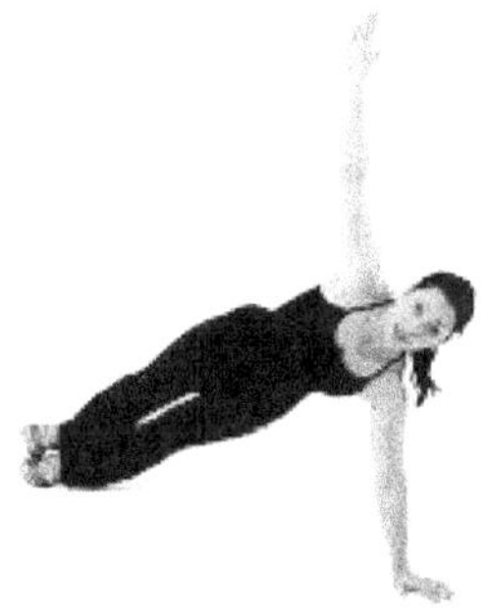

For this one begin the exercise on your knees and then with your hands beneath each shoulder, and keep your body in line from knees to head. Now bend your elbows, and keep them to the side, so that you can lower your chest all the way to the floor. Finally just straighten your arms, push yourself back up again, and then make a rising motion with your arm. Now keeping your arms straight, lift them over your head, and roll your core over to the left-hand side. Lower now and then simply rinse wash and repeat that bad boy!

T-Stand Kickbacks with Rows

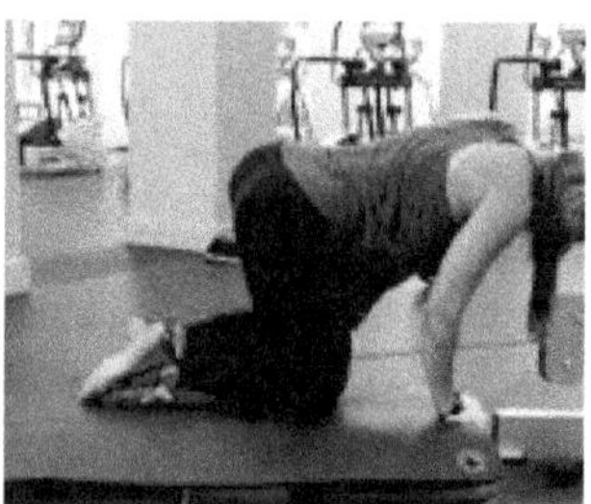

With your feet together, and with a weight in both your left and right had you can get yourself to burn a lot of calories. Now just hinge forward with your hips adjusted forward and then raise your right leg up to the back of your body. This exercise is great for strengthening your abdominal muscles while toning your gluteus maximus.

Now simply start bending your arms toward your person and by squeezing the blade of your shoulder you can then move your weights to your rib cage and begin to feel the burn! Now just press these dumbbells up and down, and then repeat the whole process again backwards for maximum effect.

Belly Flattener

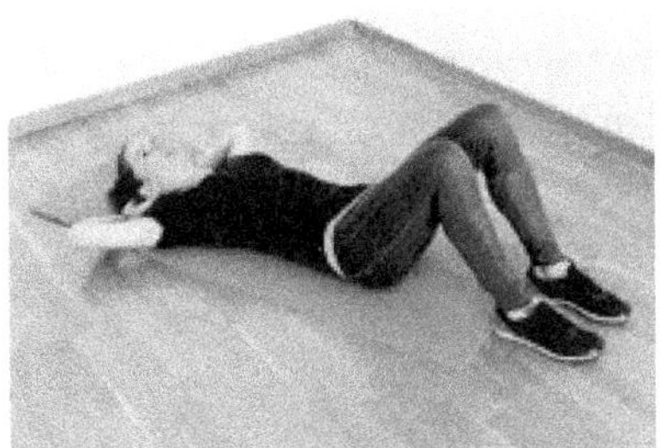

This one requires you to be a bit of a marcher. You can use this exercise to march in place for about 30 seconds. A slightly different variation of running in place, this exercise makes sure that you can take determined measured steps in order to build muscle town in your legs and in the rest of the core of your body. Do this one simple exercise in order to flatten that belly and get the rest of your body in great working order!

Full Body Roll Ups

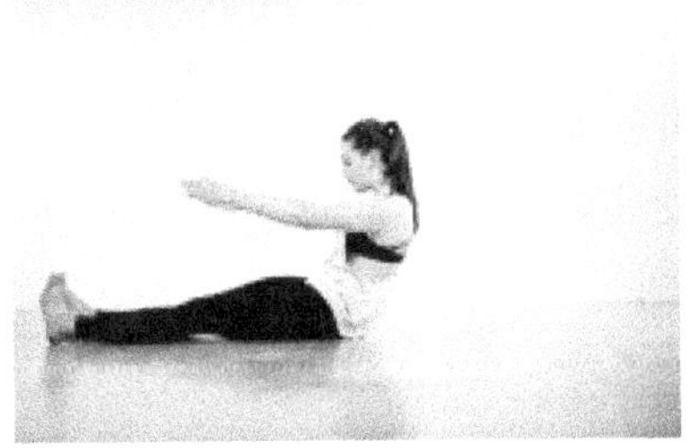

In this exercise, start out by lying on your back, extending your arms over your head. With this you can then begin to contract the muscle that runs deep inside your abdominal muscles, and then begin inhaling and raising your arms up to the ceiling. Hold this pose for just a moment.

Now let the air out of your lungs as you pull them toward the middle of your back. Finally just curl forward with your arms extended out before you. This will let you breathe in with slow controlled movements. At last you can then uncurl your body and exhale your breath at the same time. Just keep your feet to the floor as you do it. These roll ups will make you feel good in no time!

The Windmill

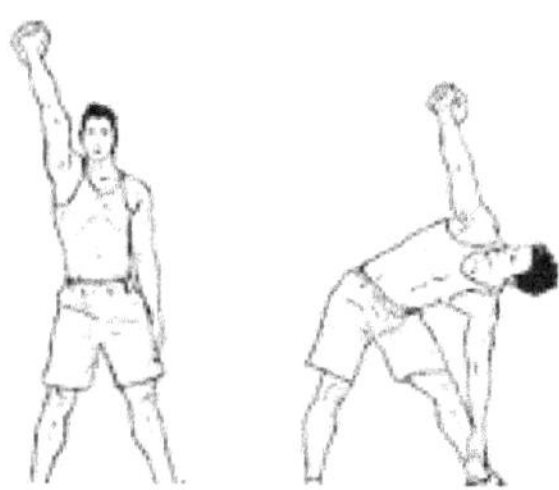

You don't have to be a Dutch windmill farmer in order to enjoy this work out! In this exercise you can have the privileged of being able to impersonate a windmill! Besides looking like an instrument of Dutch energy, you will be able to kneel with your right leg put out to your side, and your arms out with the bottoms held high. Now simply bend your core out to the left-hand side, with your left hand on the floor and raise your right up into the air, before lifting your leg up from the floor. Now just repeat the whole deal and you my friend are doing the windmill!

Crisscrosses

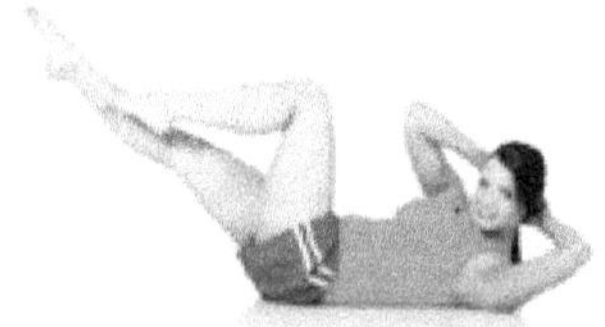

If you would like to do a crisscross, all you have to do is raise your knees up over your hips and then keep your lower legs close to the floor with your hands raised up over your head and shoulders. Now pull your neck and move up from your stomach. Like the name might imply, you are just going to do a giant crisscross maneuver in order to be able to make the most of the process. Just repeat this a few times and you will be in the best shape of your life!

Jumping Jacks

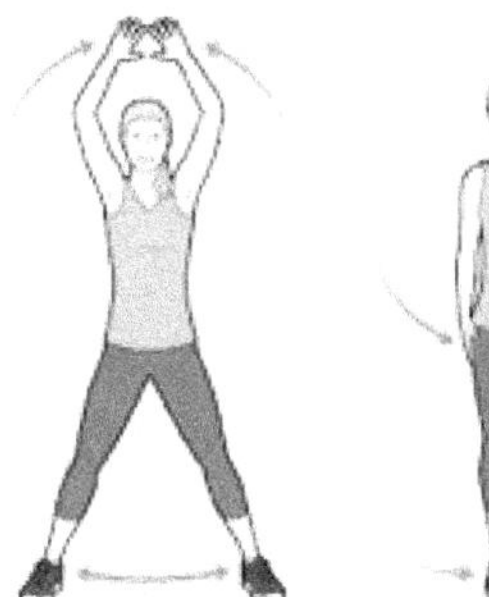

You may remember doing this at the playground during kindergarten recess. Well guess what? Jumping Jacks are still an effective means to get yourself quickly in shape! The short duration burst of energy needed in order to do Jumping Jacks is perfect for the ten minute workout. In order to do your jumping jacks, find an area in which you can extend your arms and legs all the way out. Once your body is in place, you can then just jump in the air, and extend your arms and legs out as you jump.

The Steam Engine

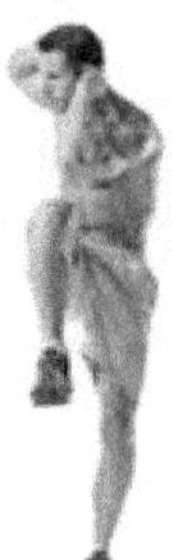

This one will roll over just like a steam engine! You will begin in a standing position and then just raise one of your knees and your elbows to get that full action work out in motion just like a locomotive rolling down the tracks! Chew! Chew! Now just do this all over again on the other side and then keep going with even more speed as you progress. This steam engine will help you stem roll right over those problem areas on your body, allowing you to streamline your whole core.

The Plank

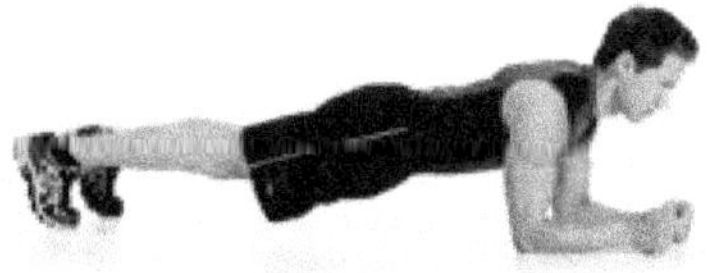

It is called the plank, because you work to make your stomach into a plank. But before you make yourself walk the plank, you first have to mold it into shape! This exercise is great for putting a little tighten up on the stomach; it launches the whole core of the body into action. It takes on the deep abdomen muscles, strengthening them in order to create a much better exercise. In order to get started o this exercise, lay right down on your face, put your arms under your shoulders and rise up until you are get right on your back.

It really doesn't get much better than this incredibly brief exercise. This exercise really works the core of your body and in order to get the most of it, you should be able to pull your bellybutton in to your back with both of your hands in sync with your shoulders. Just make sure that you keep your hips straight and hands on the ground and you will be working this one out in no time.

Running in Place

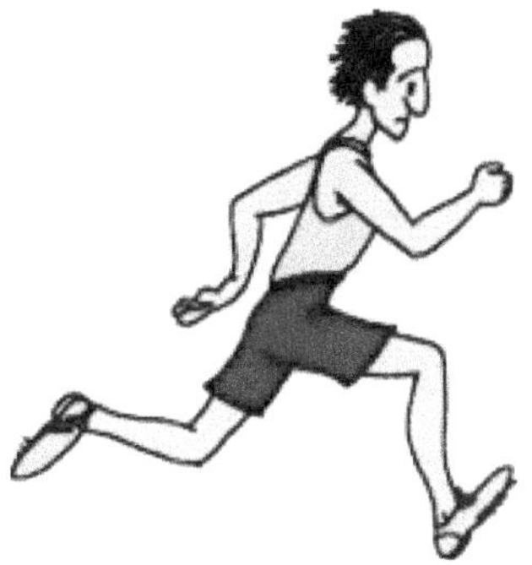

You can easily run in place and burn up a ton of calories! When I was in a college dorm room, I used to use this one workout routine to stay in shape, even in the cramped confines of the dorm. The brilliance of this simple exercise is that it can be done just about anywhere. Use this workout in order to get your legs into shape. This one is fairly simple. Just run in the same spot that you are standing in! This one will get you in shape in just ten minutes time by working your thighs, gluteus maximus, and calves! A great way to stay fit, just by running in place!

Conclusion: All in a Day's Work-out!

It can be said that exercise is half physical and half mental. And the first half of the effort most follow suite with the last half. Because if you are not mentally determined to get the job done, there is no way that you are going to be physically able to achieve the task. But once you get your mind behind your physical effort, you will be able to allow the rest to follow. Once you are mentally prepped and physically prepared, you then need to find a way to cram enough effective exercising maneuvers into your precious time schedule.

This is way short burst, high intensity training regimens are so important. You will be able to get a lot done in a short amount of time. This way you can get a great workout without cramping your style or killing the rest of your schedule. So whether you are working out at just ten minute intervals or you are doing something more, it won't overflow into your other daily activities. After completing your 10 minute interval workout regimen, you can then truly say; it was all in a day's workout!

FREE Bonus Reminder

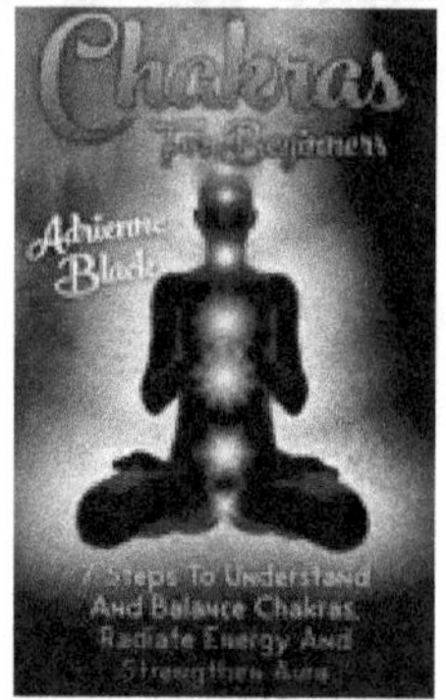

If you have not grabbed it yet, please go ahead and download your special bonus E book *"Chakras for Beginners. 7 Steps To Understand And Balance Chakras, Radiate Energy, And Strengthen Aura"*.

Simply Click the Button Below

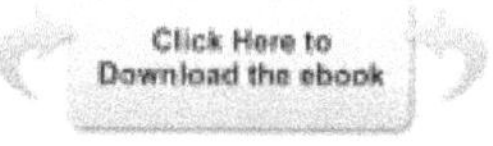

OR Go to This Page

http://lifehacksworld.com/free

BONUS #2: More Free & Discounted Books & Products

Do you want to receive more Free/Discounted Books or Products?

We have a mailing list where we send out our new Books or Products when they go free or with a discount on Amazon. Click on the link below to sign up for Free & Discount Book & Product Promotions.

=> Sign Up for Free & Discount Book & Product Promotions <=

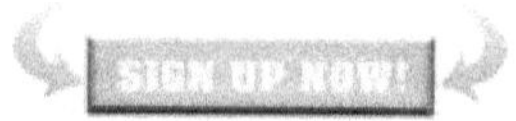

OR Go to this URL

http://zbit.ly/1WBb1Ek